BLOOD TYPE
B-POSITIVE DIET BOOK

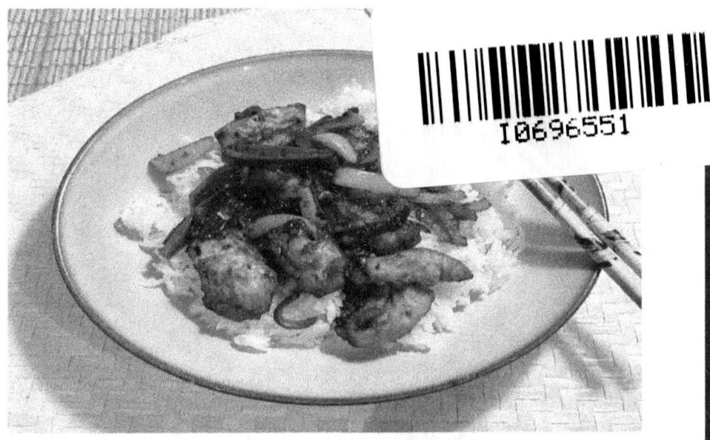

"100+ Delectable and Simple Recipes for Optimal Wellness and Long-term Health are Included in The Complete Cookbook for Your Blood Type"

Dayna G. Murphy

November 2023

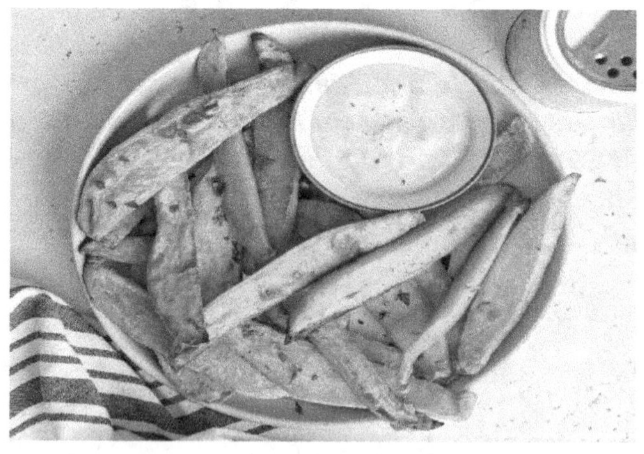

Table of Contents

INTRODUCTION 5

CHAPTER 1 7

Understanding the Diet for Blood Type B+ 7

The Advantages of Eating According to Your Blood Type 8

Tips for a Successful Blood Type B+ Diet 9

Kitchen Essentials for People with Blood Type B+ 10

CHAPTER 2 13

BLOOD TYPE B+ RECOMMENDED FOODS 13

1. GRAINS AND CEREALS 13

2. MEAT AND POULTRY 14

3. DIARY AND EGGS 14

4. SEAFOODS 15

5. NUTS AND SEEDS.. 16

6. BEVERAGES, TEAS AND COFFEE 17

7. FRUITS 17

8. HERBS AND SPICES 18

9. VEGETABLES 19

10. OILS AND FATS 20

11. BEANS AND LEGUMES 20

CHAPTER 3 .... **22**

RECIPES AND INGREDIENTS 22

10 Breakfast Delights 22

10 Wholesome Lunches 29

10 Delectable Dinners 38

10 Snacks and Sides 46

10 Sweet Treats 53

10 Beverages 59

Conclusion **67**

Journals to Plan Your Diet **70**

INTRODUCTION

Janet was a buddy of mine once upon a time. She had a B+ blood type and was always looking for nutritious foods. Janet tried the dishes in my *Blood Type B+ Diet Cookbook*, and they changed her life. She felt more energized, her digestion improved, and she even lost some weight.

Seeing Janet benefit from the cookbook prompted me to write and spread the word about the proper diet. I wanted to help others discover the correct foods for their blood types, as Janet had. It felt amazing to know that anything I made a difference in her health and well-being.

Janet's experience with the Blood Type B+ diet demonstrated the power of eating appropriately for your blood type, and it inspired me to share this knowledge with additional people so that they, too, could benefit from a personalized and healthy diet.

The **"Blood Type B+ Diet:** Nourishing Your Body, Your Way." This thorough book is your key to living a happier, more vibrant life by tailoring your diet to your specific blood type. This book delves into the complexities of the Blood

Type B+ diet, which is designed exclusively for people with this blood type.

You'll find a wide choice of delicious and nutritionally-balanced dishes that adapt to your unique needs, thanks to well-researched insights and expert recommendations. This book presents a holistic approach to eating that complements your blood type, from lean proteins to full grains, fresh veggies, and delicious sweet indulgences.

Whether you want to enhance your overall health, increase your energy, or lose weight, the Blood Type B+ Diet book gives you the knowledge and skills to make smart nutritional decisions. It's time to go on a well-being journey that is personally suited to you, and this book is your trusted companion on that journey to a better and happier self.

CHAPTER 1

Understanding the Diet for Blood Type B+

The Blood Type B+ diet is a diet based on the blood type diet ideas promoted by a scientist. Individuals with Blood Type B+ (or B positive) should consume specific foods that fit with their blood type to achieve optimal health and well-being, according to this diet.

The Blood Type B+ diet idea proposes that people with this blood type may have distinct genetic and digestive features that influence how their bodies react to various foods. As a result, adapting one's diet to one's blood type may improve general health and help prevent a variety of health problems.

The following are common Blood Type B+ diet components:

1. Foods to Focus on: People with Blood Type B+ are often advised to have a well-balanced diet rich in lean meats, dairy, seafood, fruits, and vegetables. Specific foods, such as lamb, mutton, and green vegetables, are thought to be tolerated well.

Avoid foods such as poultry, corn, peanuts, and tomatoes, which are thought to be less friendly with this blood type.

2. Individual Differences: It's vital to understand that not everyone with the same blood type has the same dietary requirements. Each person is unique, and when following this diet, aspects such as heredity, lifestyle, and overall health must be taken into account.

The Advantages of Eating According to Your Blood Type

Proponents of the Blood Type B+ diet claim that following this specific eating plan can provide various potential benefits:

1. Better Digestion: Eating foods that are suitable with your blood type may result in improved digestion and nutrient absorption, lowering the chance of digestive discomfort.

2. Enhanced Energy: According to the diet, eating in accordance with your blood type will boost energy levels and overall vitality.

3. Weight control: Some people say the Blood Type B+ diet helps with weight control and loss since it promotes a balanced and individualized approach to nutrition.

4. Reduced Risk of Chronic Diseases: Proponents think that by avoiding foods that may be less compatible with your blood type, you can lower your risk of certain health disorders, while scientific evidence to support this claim is lacking.

Tips for a Successful Blood Type B+ Diet

Here are some recommendations to help you succeed if you are considering or are already following the Blood Type B+ diet:

1. Consult a Healthcare practitioner: Before making major dietary changes, speak with a healthcare practitioner or registered dietitian. They can provide you tailored advice and make sure your food choices are safe and balanced.

2. Plan Your Meals: Make a weekly diet plan that includes a variety of Blood Type B+ suitable foods. This can help you keep on track and maintain a well-balanced diet.

3. Examine Food Labels: Examine food labels carefully to detect components that may be incompatible with your blood type. Avoid chemicals and preservatives in processed meals.

4. Pay Attention to Your Body: While the diet provides suggestions, pay attention to how your body reacts to various foods. Everyone is different, and everyone's tolerance differs.

Kitchen Essentials for People with Blood Type B+

It's helpful to have a well-equipped kitchen to supplement your Blood Type B+ diet. Here are a few things to think about:

1. Quality Knives: Invest in sharp, high-quality knives for slicing, dicing, and chopping your fresh veggies and meats.

2. Food Processor: A food processor can speed up meal preparation, especially for recipes that call for finely chopped or pureed components.

3. Cookware: For healthier cooking with less oil or butter, use nonstick pots and pans. A decent set of stainless steel cookware is also a worthwhile investment.

4. Blender: A strong blender is required for creating fresh smoothies and soups.

5. Food Storage Containers: To keep your Blood Type B+ compatible ingredients fresh, invest in a range of food storage containers.

6. Steamer: Steaming is a healthy cooking method, and a vegetable steamer may help you conveniently prepare a variety of vegetables.

7. Spices and herbs: Using a well-stocked spice rack, you may add flavor to your foods without using hazardous additives.

8. Cutting Boards: To prevent cross-contamination, use separate cutting boards for different types of ingredients (e.g., one for meat and one for veggies).

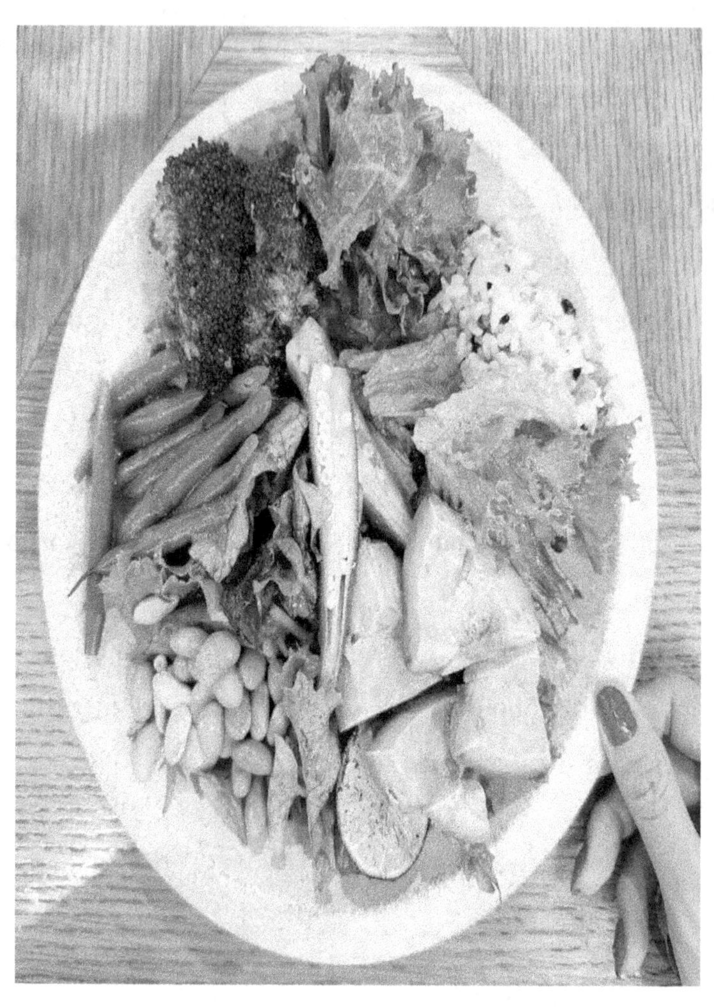

CHAPTER 2

BLOOD TYPE B+ RECOMMENDED FOODS

1. GRAINS AND CEREALS

Grain/Cereal	Portion Size	Frequency per Week
Brown Rice	1/2 to 1 cup cooked	2-4 times
Oatmeal (Steel-Cut)	1/2 to 1 cup cooked	2-3 times
Millet	1/2 to 1 cup cooked	1-2 times
Quinoa	1/2 to 1 cup cooked	2-4 times
Spelt	1/2 to 1 cup cooked	2-3 times
Amaranth	1/2 to 1 cup cooked	1-2 times
Buckwheat	1/2 to 1 cup cooked	2-3 times

Barley	1/2 to 1 cup cooked	1-2 times
Rye	1/2 to 1 cup cooked	1-2 times
Teff	1/2 to 1 cup cooked	2-3 times

2. MEAT AND POULTRY

Meat/Poultry	Portion Size	Frequency per Week
Lamb	3-4 ounces (cooked)	2-3 times
Venison	3-4 ounces (cooked)	2-3 times
Rabbit	3-4 ounces (cooked)	1-2 times

3. DIARY AND EGGS

Dairy/Eggs	Portion Size	Frequency per Week
Eggs	2-4 eggs per week	2-3 times

Yogurt (plain)	1/2 to 1 cup	2-4 times
Kefir	1/2 to 1 cup	2-4 times
Goat Cheese	1 ounce	2-3 times

4. SEAFOODS

Seafood	Portion Size	Frequency per Week
Mahi-Mahi	4-6 ounces (cooked)	2-3 times
Halibut	4-6 ounces (cooked)	2-3 times
Cod	4-6 ounces (cooked)	2-3 times
Salmon	4-6 ounces (cooked)	2-4 times
Trout	4-6 ounces (cooked)	2-3 times
Mackerel	4-6 ounces (cooked)	1-2 times
Sardines	4-6 ounces (cooked)	1-2 times

| Flounder | 4-6 ounces (cooked) | 2-3 times |

5. NUTS AND SEEDS

Nuts/Seeds	Portion Size	Frequency per Week
Almonds	1 ounce (about 23 nuts)	3-4 times
Walnuts	1 ounce (about 14 halves)	3-4 times
Flaxseeds (ground)	1-2 tablespoons	2-3 times
Chia Seeds	1-2 tablespoons	2-3 times
Pine Nuts	1 ounce (about 167 nuts)	2-3 times
Sesame Seeds	1-2 tablespoons	2-3 times
Pumpkin Seeds	1 ounce (about 85 seeds)	2-3 times
Sunflower Seeds	1 ounce (about 87 seeds)	2-3 times

6. BEVERAGES, TEAS AND COFFEE

Beverage/Tea/ Coffee	Portion Size	Frequency per Week
Green Tea	1-2 cups	2-4 times
Peppermint Tea	1-2 cups	2-3 times
Ginseng Tea	1-2 cups	2-3 times
Licorice Tea	1-2 cups	2-3 times
Coffee (if desired)	1-2 cups	Occasional
Water	8-10 glasses (8 oz each)	Daily
Herbal Infusions (e.g., chamomile, ginger)	1-2 cups	2-3 times

7. FRUITS

Fruit	Portion Size	Frequency per Week
Plums	1 medium or 1 cup	3-4 times

Cherries	1 cup	3-4 times
Pineapple	1 cup	2-3 times
Papaya	1 cup	2-3 times
Grapes	1 cup	2-3 times
Cranberries	1 cup	2-3 times
Watermelon	1 cup	2-3 times
Figs	2 medium or 1/2 cup	2-3 times

8. HERBS AND SPICES

Herbs/Spices	Portion Size	Frequency per Week
Ginger	1-2 teaspoons (freshly grated)	3-4 times
Turmeric	1-2 teaspoons (ground)	3-4 times
Parsley	1-2 teaspoons (freshly chopped)	2-3 times
Rosemary	1-2 teaspoons (fresh or dried)	2-3 times

Thyme	1-2 teaspoons (fresh or dried)	2-3 times
Cilantro (Coriander)	1-2 teaspoons (freshly chopped)	2-3 times
Dill	1-2 teaspoons (freshly chopped)	2-3 times
Mint	1-2 teaspoons (freshly chopped)	2-3 times

9. VEGETABLES

Vegetable	Portion Size	Frequency per Week
Spinach	1 cup (cooked)	3-4 times
Kale	1 cup (cooked)	3-4 times
Broccoli	1 cup (cooked)	2-3 times
Brussels Sprouts	1 cup (cooked)	2-3 times
Sweet Potatoes	1 medium	2-3 times
Carrots	1 medium	2-3 times

| Red Peppers | 1 medium | 2-3 times |
| Beetroot | 1 medium | 2-3 times |

10. OILS AND FATS

Oil/Fat	Portion Size	Frequency per Week
Olive Oil	1-2 tablespoons	3-4 times
Flaxseed Oil	1-2 teaspoons	2-3 times
Walnut Oil	1-2 teaspoons	2-3 times
Ghee (Clarified Butter)	1-2 teaspoons	2-3 times
Almond Butter	1-2 tablespoons	2-3 times
Avocado	1/4 to 1/2 avocado	3-4 times
Coconut Oil	1-2 tablespoons	1-2 times

11. BEANS AND LEGUMES

Beans/Legumes	Portion Size	Frequency per Week
Black-Eyed Peas	1/2 to 1 cup cooked	2-3 times
Pinto Beans	1/2 to 1 cup cooked	2-3 times
Red Lentils	1/2 to 1 cup cooked	2-3 times
Green Lentils	1/2 to 1 cup cooked	2-3 times
Black Beans	1/2 to 1 cup cooked	2-3 times
Garbanzo Beans (Chickpeas)	1/2 to 1 cup cooked	2-3 times
Navy Beans	1/2 to 1 cup cooked	2-3 times
Adzuki Beans	1/2 to 1 cup cooked	2-3 times

CHAPTER 3

RECIPES AND INGREDIENTS

10 Breakfast Delights

1. Spinach and Feta Scrambled Eggs

Ingredients:

- 2 eggs
- 1 cup fresh spinach - 1/4 cup crumbled feta cheese
- Season with salt and pepper to taste

Instructions:

1. In a small saucepan over medium heat, heat a tiny amount of olive oil.

2. Add the spinach and cook until wilted.

3. Whisk the eggs in a mixing dish and season with salt and pepper.

4. Add the eggs and wilted spinach to the pan.

5. Cook until the eggs are scrambled, stirring periodically.

6. Sprinkle with feta cheese and heat for another minute.

7. Serve immediately.

(Preparation time: 10 minutes)

2. Blueberry Buckwheat Pancakes

Ingredients:

- 1 cup buckwheat flour 1 cup fresh blueberries
- 1 tablespoon almond milk
- 1/2 teaspoon baking powder - 1 egg
- 1 teaspoon honey
- Extra virgin olive oil

Instructions:

1. Combine the buckwheat flour and baking powder in a mixing dish.

2. Combine the egg, almond milk, and honey in a mixing bowl. Mix until everything is well blended.

3. Fold in the blueberries gently.

4. In a skillet over medium heat, heat the olive oil.

5. Ladle a ladle of batter onto the skillet and cook until bubbles appear on the surface.

6. Cook until both sides of the pancake are brown.

7. Continue with the remaining batter. Serve with more blueberries and honey.

(Preparation time: 20 minutes)

3. Honey and Almond Greek Yogurt Parfait

Ingredients:

- 1 cup plain Greek yogurt

- 1 teaspoon honey

- 1/4 cup almonds, sliced

- Fresh berries (strawberries, blueberries, etc.)

Instructions:

1. Layer Greek yogurt, honey, almonds, and fresh berries in a glass or bowl.

2. Continue layering as desired.

3. Enjoy this simple and healthy parfait.

(Preparation time: 5 minutes)

3. Quinoa Breakfast Bowl with Fresh Fruit

Ingredients:

- 1/2 cup cooked quinoa - Banana, strawberry, and kiwi slices

- Chopped nuts (almonds, walnuts, etc.)

- Drizzling honey or maple syrup

Instructions:

1. Cook the quinoa according to package directions and set aside to cool.

2. Place cooked quinoa in a mixing basin.

3. Garnish with fresh fruit slices and chopped nuts.

4. Drizzle the bowl with honey or maple syrup.

5. Stir everything together and enjoy a nutritious breakfast.

(Preparation time: 15 minutes)

5. Kale and Kiwi Green Smoothie

Ingredients:

- 1 cup kale greens - 2 peeled and sliced kiwis
- 1/2 cup plain Greek yogurt
- Half a cup almond milk
- 1 teaspoon honey
- Cubes of ice

Instructions:

1. In a blender, combine kale, kiwis, Greek yogurt, almond milk, honey, and ice cubes.

2. Puree until smooth.

3. Serve your cool green smoothie in a glass.

(Preparation time: 10 minutes)

6. Soup with Lentils and Vegetables

Ingredients:

- 1/2 cup chopped tomatoes - 1 cup cooked lentils - 1 cup mixed vegetables (carrots, bell peppers, zucchini)

- 1 tablespoon olive oil
- Season with salt and pepper to taste

Instructions:

1. Heat the olive oil in a saucepan over medium heat.

2. Add the mixed vegetables and sauté until tender.

3. Combine cooked lentils and diced tomatoes in a mixing bowl.

4. Adjust the soup consistency with water or veggie broth to taste.

5. Season with salt and pepper and continue to cook until heated through.

6. Serve immediately for a flavorful breakfast.

(Preparation time: 15 minutes)

7. Fresh Fruit Quinoa Breakfast Bowl

Ingredients:

- 1/2 cup cooked quinoa - Banana, strawberry, and kiwi slices
- Chopped nuts (almonds, walnuts, etc.)
- Drizzling honey or maple syrup

Instructions:

1. Cook the quinoa according to package directions and set aside to cool.

2. Place cooked quinoa in a mixing basin.

3. Garnish with fresh fruit slices and chopped nuts.

4. Drizzle the bowl with honey or maple syrup.

5. Stir everything together and enjoy a nutritious breakfast.

(Preparation time: 15 minutes)

8. Salad with Avocado and Shrimp

Ingredients:

- half an avocado, sliced
- 6 to 8 cooked shrimp
- Mixed greens (spinach, arugula, etc.)
- Tomatoes, cherry
- Dressing: olive oil and lemon juice
- Season with salt and pepper to taste

Instructions:

1. Arrange a platter with mixed greens.

2. Arrange sliced avocado, cooked shrimp, and cherry tomatoes on top.

3. Drizzle with lemon juice and olive oil.

4. Season to taste with salt and pepper.

5. Start your day with a light, protein-packed breakfast salad.
(Preparation time: 10 minutes)

9. Cumin-Spiced Sweet Potato Fries

Ingredients:

- 1 medium sweet potato, cut into fries

Instructions:

1. Preheat the oven to 425 degrees Fahrenheit (220 degrees Celsius).
2. Combine sweet potato fries, olive oil, cumin, salt, and pepper in a mixing bowl.
3. Spread out on a baking sheet.
4. Bake the fries for 20-25 minutes, or until crispy.
5. Serve immediately.
(Preparation time: 30 minutes, plus baking time)

10. Chia Seed Pudding with Berries

Ingredients:

- 2 teaspoons chia seeds
- Half a cup almond milk
- 1/2 teaspoon vanilla essence - mixed berries (blueberries, raspberries) - honey drizzle

Instructions:

1. Combine chia seeds, almond milk, and vanilla extract in a jar or container.

2. Stir thoroughly and place in the refrigerator for at least 2 hours or overnight, until thickened.

3. Garnish with mixed berries and honey drizzle.

4. Have a nutritious chia seed pudding for breakfast.

(Preparation time: 2 hours or overnight soaking)

10 Wholesome Lunches

1. Salad with grilled chicken and vegetables

Ingredients:

- Chicken breast grilled
- Mixed greens (spinach, arugula, etc.)
- Tomatoes in the shape of cherries
- Cucumber slices
- Dressing: olive oil and balsamic vinegar
- Season with salt and pepper to taste.

Instructions:

1. Grill the chicken breast until it is completely done.
2. Chicken should be cut into strips.

3. On a platter, arrange mixed greens.

4. Top with grilled chicken, cherry tomatoes, and cucumbers.

5. Drizzle with balsamic vinegar and olive oil.

6. Season with salt and pepper to taste.

7. Eat a protein-rich salad.

(Preparation time: 20 minutes)

2. Bowl of Quinoa with Black Beans

Ingredients:

- Quinoa has been cooked.

- canned or cooked black beans

- Avocado slices

- fresh cilantro, chopped

- Juice of lime

- To taste, drizzle with olive oil and season with salt and pepper.

Instructions:

1. Combine cooked quinoa and black beans in a mixing basin.

2. Add sliced avocado and cilantro to taste.

3. Drizzle with olive oil and lime juice.

4. Season with salt and pepper to taste.

5. Stir everything together and serve a hearty quinoa bowl.

(Preparation time: 15 minutes)

3. Hummus-topped Greek Salad

- *Ingredients:*
- Mixed greens (for example, Romaine lettuce)
- Tomatoes in the shape of cherries
- Slices of cucumber
- Slices of red onion
- The Kalamata olives
- Feta is a type of cheese.
- Hummus (dipped or dressed)

Instructions:

1. On a platter, arrange mixed greens.

2. Add cherry tomatoes, cucumber, red onion, Kalamata olives, and feta cheese to the top.

3. Serve with hummus on the side or sprinkle with olive oil as a dressing.

4. Enjoy a light, Mediterranean-inspired salad.

(Preparation time: 15 minutes)

4. Asparagus and salmon

- *Ingredients:*
- Fillet of salmon
- Asparagus spears, fresh
- Lemon juice and olive oil
- Dill, freshly picked
- Season with salt and pepper to taste.

Instructions:

1. Preheat the oven to 400 degrees Fahrenheit (200 degrees Celsius).
2. On a baking sheet, place the fish and asparagus.
3. Drizzle with lemon juice and olive oil.
4. Season with fresh dill, salt, and pepper to taste.
5. Bake for 15-20 minutes, or until the fish readily flakes.
6. Serve hot for a filling, tasty supper.

(Preparation time: 25 minutes)

5. Stir-Fry of Lentils and Vegetables

Ingredients:

- Lentils are cooked lentils.
- Vegetable stir-fry (e.g., bell peppers, broccoli, snap peas)
- Extra virgin olive oil
- Tamari or soy sauce
- minced fresh ginger and garlic
- Optional crushed red pepper flakes

Instructions:

1. Warm the olive oil in a pan over medium-high heat.
2. Sauté for a minute with the minced ginger and garlic.
3. Cook until the mixed vegetables are soft.
4. Cooked lentils, soy sauce, and red pepper flakes (if using) should be added now.
5. Stir-fry until well hot.
6. Serve for a nutritious and filling lunch.

(Preparation time: 20 minutes)

6. Wrap with turkey and avocado

Ingredients:

- Wrap or tortilla made from whole grains
- turkey breast, sliced

- Avocado slices
- Greens, mixed
- Optional Dijon mustard
- Season with salt and pepper to taste.

Instructions:

1. Place the whole-grain wrap or tortilla on a plate.
2. Layer sliced turkey, avocado, and mixed greens on top.
3. If preferred, season with Dijon mustard.
4. Season with salt and pepper to taste.
5. Roll the wrap up and cut it in half.
6. Enjoy a quick and tasty lunch.

(Preparation time: 10 minutes)

7. Green Salad with Tuna

Ingredients:

- Tuna in water, canned
- Greens (arugula, baby spinach, etc.)
- Tomatoes in the shape of cherries
- Cucumber slices
- Dressing: balsamic vinaigrette
- Season with salt and pepper to taste.

Instructions:

1. Combine canned tuna (drained) and mixed greens in a mixing basin.

2. Add cherry tomatoes and cucumber slices.

3. Dress with the balsamic vinaigrette.

4. Season with salt and pepper to taste.

5. Toss everything together and serve a protein-packed salad.

(Preparation time: 10 minutes)

8. Stir-Fry with Vegetables and Quinoa

Ingredients:

- Quinoa has been cooked.
- Vegetable stir-fry (e.g., bell peppers, broccoli, snap peas)
- Extra virgin olive oil
- Tamari or soy sauce
- minced fresh ginger and garlic
- Optional crushed red pepper flakes

Instructions:

1. Warm the olive oil in a pan over medium-high heat.

2. Sauté for a minute with the minced ginger and garlic.

3. Cook until the mixed vegetables are soft.

4. Cooked quinoa, soy sauce, and red pepper flakes (if using) should be added now.

5. Stir-fry until well hot.

6. Serve for a nutritious and filling lunch.

(Preparation time: 20 minutes)

9. Stir-Fry with Chicken and Vegetables

Ingredients:

- sliced chicken breast or thigh
- Vegetable stir-fry (e.g., bell peppers, broccoli, snap peas)
- Extra virgin olive oil
- Tamari or soy sauce
- minced fresh ginger and garlic
- Optional crushed red pepper flakes

Instructions:

1. Warm the olive oil in a pan over medium-high heat.

2. Sauté for a minute with the minced ginger and garlic.

3. Cook until the cut chicken is no longer pink.

4. Cook until the mixed vegetables are soft.

5. Drizzle with soy sauce and, if using, red pepper flakes.

6. Stir-fry until well hot.

7. Serve hot for a filling and protein-rich lunch.

(Preparation time: 20 minutes)

10. Salad with Sweet Potatoes and Chickpeas

Ingredients:

- Cubes of roasted sweet potato
- Chickpeas (cooked or canned)
- Greens (such as kale and spinach)
- Red onions, sliced
- Dressing with olive oil and lemon juice
- Season with salt and pepper to taste.

Instructions:

1. Combine the roasted sweet potato, chickpeas, and mixed greens in a mixing basin.

2. Serve with chopped red onions.

3. Drizzle with lemon juice and olive oil.

4. Season with salt and pepper to taste.

5. Toss everything together and serve a substantial and tasty salad.

(Preparation time: 15 minutes)

10 Delectable Dinners

1. Lemon and Dill Baked Salmon

Ingredients:

- Salmon fillets - Dill leaves - Lemon slices - Olive oil
- Season with salt and pepper to taste

Instructions:

1. Preheat the oven to 375 degrees Fahrenheit (190 degrees Celsius).

2. Line a baking sheet with salmon fillets.

3. Season with salt and pepper and drizzle with olive oil.

4. Garnish with dill and lemon slices.

5. Bake for 15-20 minutes, or until the fish readily flakes.

6. Serve immediately. (Preparation time: 25 minutes)

2. Stir-Fry of Quinoa and Vegetables

Ingredients:

- Quinoa cooked - Stir-fried vegetables (e.g., bell peppers, broccoli, snap peas)

- Extra virgin olive oil
- Tamari or soy sauce
- Minced fresh ginger and garlic
- Optional crushed red pepper flakes

Instructions:

1. Heat the olive oil in a pan over medium-high heat.

2. Cook for a minute after adding the minced ginger and garlic.

3. Cook until the mixed vegetables are soft.

4. Stir in the cooked quinoa, soy sauce, and (if using) red pepper flakes.

5. Stir-fry until well cooked.

6. Serve hot for a nutritious and filling dinner.

(Preparation time: 20 minutes)

3. Chickpea Salad from the Mediterranean

Ingredients:

- Drained canned chickpeas - Halved cherry tomatoes
- Cucumber and red onion slices
- Kalamata olives - Feta cheese - Dressing of olive oil and balsamic vinegar - Fresh basil leaves
- Season with salt and pepper to taste

Instructions:

1. Combine chickpeas, cherry tomatoes, cucumber, red onion, Kalamata olives, and feta cheese in a mixing bowl.

2. Drizzle with balsamic vinegar and olive oil.

3. Tear fresh basil leaves into the salad and toss them in.

4. Season with salt and pepper to taste.

5. Toss everything together and serve a tasty Mediterranean dinner.

(Preparation time: 15 minutes)

4. Skewers with grilled turkey and vegetables

Ingredients:

- Cubed turkey breast or thigh -Cubed bell peppers, zucchini, and red onion
- Lemon juice - Olive oil
- Thyme or rosemary, fresh
- Season with salt and pepper to taste

Instructions:

1. Get your grill or grill pan ready.

2. Make skewers by alternately skewering turkey and veggies.

3. Drizzle with lemon juice and olive oil.

4. Garnish with thyme or rosemary.

5. Season with salt and pepper to taste.

6. Grill for 10-15 minutes, turning regularly, until the turkey is cooked through and the veggies are soft.

7. Serve immediately for a delectable grilled supper.

(Preparation time: 30 minutes)

5. Vegetable and Lentil Soup

Ingredients:

- Diced tomatoes - Cooked lentils - Mixed veggies (carrots, bell peppers, zucchini) - Olive oil
- Thyme or rosemary, fresh
- Season with salt and pepper to taste

Instructions:

1. Heat the olive oil in a saucepan over medium heat.

2. Add the mixed vegetables and sauté until tender.

3. Combine cooked lentils and diced tomatoes in a mixing bowl.

4. Adjust the soup consistency with water or veggie broth to taste.

5. Add fresh thyme or rosemary, salt, and pepper to taste.

6. Simmer until well heated.

7. Serve immediately for a filling and nutritious dinner.

(Preparation time: 25 minutes)

6. Sweet Potatoes with Roasted Chicken

Ingredients:

- Thighs or breasts of chicken
- Cubed sweet potato - Olive oil - Paprika - Cumin
- Season with salt and pepper to taste

Instructions:

1. Preheat the oven to 400 degrees Fahrenheit (200 degrees Celsius).

2. Line a baking sheet with chicken and sweet potato pieces.

3. Finish with a drizzle of olive oil.

4. Season with paprika, cumin, salt, and pepper to taste.

5. Roast for 25-30 minutes, or until the chicken is cooked through and the sweet potatoes are soft.

6. Serve immediately.

(Preparation time: 35 minutes)

7. Stir-Fry of Vegetables and Tofu

Ingredients:

- Cubed extra-firm tofu - Stir-fry vegetables (broccoli, snap peas, carrots)

- Extra virgin olive oil

- Tamari or soy sauce

- Minced fresh ginger and garlic

- Optional crushed red pepper flakes

Instructions:

1. Heat the olive oil in a pan over medium-high heat.

2. Cook for a minute after adding the minced ginger and garlic.

3. Cook until the mixed vegetables are soft.

4. Stir in the tofu cubes, soy sauce, and red pepper flakes (if using).

5. Stir-fry until well cooked.

6. Serve hot for a nutritious and filling dinner.

(Preparation time: 25 minutes)

8. Pesto Spaghetti Squash

Ingredients:

- Spaghetti squash - Pesto sauce, homemade or store-bought

- Halved cherry tomatoes - Fresh basil leaves - Grated Parmesan cheese

- Season with salt and pepper to taste

Instructions:

1. Preheat the oven to 375 degrees Fahrenheit (190 degrees Celsius).

2. Split the spaghetti squash in half lengthwise and scoop out the seeds.

3. Arrange the squash on a baking sheet, cut side down.

4. Bake for 30-40 minutes, or until the squash is soft and readily shredded with a fork.

5. Toss the squash strands with the pesto sauce.

6. Garnish with cherry tomatoes, fresh basil, and Parmesan cheese.

7. Season with salt and pepper to taste.

8. Serve as a tasty low-carb meal.

(Preparation time: 50 minutes)

9. Lettuce Wraps with Turkey and Avocado

Ingredients:

- Ground turkey - Lettuce (iceberg, Romaine) - Sliced avocado

- Tomatoes, diced

- Salsa (optional) - Fresh cilantro leaves

- Season with salt and pepper to taste

Instructions:

1. Brown and completely cook ground turkey in a skillet.

2. Season with salt and pepper to taste.

3. Fill lettuce wraps with turkey, avocado slices, diced tomatoes, fresh cilantro, and salsa (if using).

4. Roll up the lettuce leaves and serve for a light, low-carb meal.

(Preparation time: 20 minutes)

10. Stuffed Eggplant and Tomato Peppers

Ingredients:

- Halved and seeded bell peppers - Diced eggplant - Diced tomatoes

- Chopped onion - Olive oil - Fresh basil and oregano - Season with salt and pepper to taste

Instructions:

1. Preheat the oven to 375 degrees Fahrenheit (190 degrees Celsius).

2. Heat the olive oil in a pan over medium heat.

3. Cook until the onion and eggplant are soft.

4. Add the chopped tomatoes and fresh herbs and mix well.

5. Season with salt and pepper to taste.

Fill the bell pepper halves halfway with the eggplant-tomato mixture.

Cover with foil and place in a baking dish.

8. Bake for 30-40 minutes, or until the peppers are tender.

9. Serve immediately for a tasty vegetarian supper.

(Preparation time: 45 minutes)

10 Snacks and Sides

1. Hummus and Veggie Sticks

Ingredients:

- Hummus (purchased or homemade)
- Sticks of carrot
- Carrot sticks
- Slices of bell pepper

Instructions:

1. Wash the vegetables and chop them into sticks.

2. Serve with hummus on the side for dipping.

3. Snack on something quick and healthful.

(Preparation time: 10 minutes)

2. Berries in Greek Yogurt

Ingredients:

- Yogurt from Greece
- Fresh berries (blueberries, strawberries, and raspberries, for example)
- Honey (optional)

Instructions:

1. Place Greek yogurt in a bowl.

2. Garnish with fresh berries.

3. If desired, drizzle with honey.

4. Have a protein-rich, sweet snack.

(Preparation time: 5 minutes)

3. Salad with Cucumber and Tomatoes

Ingredients:

- Cucumber slices
- Halved cherry tomatoes
- Red onion slices
- Dressing of olive oil and balsamic vinegar
- Fresh basil leaves
- Salt and pepper to taste

Instructions:

1. Combine sliced cucumbers, cherry tomatoes, and red onion in a mixing dish.

2. Drizzle with balsamic vinegar and olive oil.

3. Tear fresh basil leaves into the salad and toss them in.

4. Season with salt and pepper to taste.

5. Toss to blend and serve as a refreshing side dish.

(Preparation time: 10 minutes)

4. Whole-Grain Tortilla Chips with Guacamole

Ingredients:

- Diced tomatoes
- Chopped red onion
- Fresh cilantro leaves
- Lime juice
- Season with salt and pepper to taste
- Serve with whole-grain tortilla chips

Instructions:

1. In a mixing bowl, mash ripe avocados.

2. Fold in the diced tomatoes, red onion, and fresh cilantro.

3. Squeeze lime juice over the top of the mixture.

4. Season with salt and pepper to taste.

5. Serve with whole-grain tortilla chips as a dip.

6. Snack on something creamy and flavorful.

(Preparation time: 15 minutes)

5. Edamame Steamed

Ingredients:

- Edamame (fresh or frozen)
- Optional sea salt

Instructions:

1. Cook the edamame according to the package directions.

2. If desired, season with sea salt.

3. Serve in the pods for a high-protein snack.

4. Have a quick and healthful side dish.

(Preparation time: 5 minutes)

6. Skewers of Caprese

Ingredients:

- Fresh mozzarella balls
- Fresh basil leaves
- Balsamic glaze
- Skewers or toothpicks

Instructions:

1. Thread cherry tomatoes, mozzarella balls, and fresh basil leaves onto skewers.

2. Finish with a drizzle of balsamic glaze.

3. Serve as a delectable and simple side dish.

(Preparation time: 10 minutes)

7. Garlic-Sautéed Spinach

Ingredients:

- Minced garlic
- Olive oil
- Fresh spinach
- Season with salt and pepper to taste
- Serve with lemon wedges (optional).

Instructions:

1. Heat the olive oil in a pan over medium heat.

2. Cook for a minute after adding the minced garlic.

3. Cook until the spinach is wilted.

4. Season with salt and pepper to taste.

5. If preferred, squeeze lemon wedges over the sautéed spinach.

6. Serve as a nutritious, garlicky side dish.

(Preparation time: 10 minutes)

8. Dried Fruits and Mixed Nuts

Ingredients:

- A variety of mixed nuts (almonds, walnuts, cashews, etc.)
- Dried fruits (such as apricots and cranberries)
- Optional dark chocolate chips

Instructions:

1. In a mixing dish, combine a variety of mixed nuts and dried fruits.

2. If preferred, add dark chocolate chips for a hint of sweetness.

3. Divide into snack-sized bags for a quick on-the-go snack.

(Preparation time: 5 minutes)

9. Almond Butter Rice Cakes

Ingredients:

- Rice cakes made from whole grains
- Almond milk
- Banana slices
- Optional: honey

Instructions:

1. Spread whole-grain rice cakes with almond butter.

2. Drizzle with honey if preferred and top with sliced bananas.

3. Have a quick and filling snack.

(Preparation time: 5 minutes)

10 slices avocado and tomato

Ingredients:

- Avocado, sliced

- Tomatoes, sliced

- Olive oil,

- fresh basil leaves,

- balsamic glaze (optional),

- salt and pepper to taste

Instructions:

1. Arrange the avocado and tomato slices on a platter.

2. Drizzle with olive oil and, if desired, balsamic glaze.

3. Scatter fresh basil leaves over the slices.

4. Season with salt and pepper to taste.

5. Enjoy a light and quick side dish.

(Preparation time: 10 minutes)

10 Sweet Treats

1. Berry-Yogurt Parfait

Ingredients:

- Yogurt from Greece
- Berries (blueberries, strawberries, raspberries, etc.)
- Honey - Optional granola

Instructions:

1. Layer Greek yogurt and mixed berries in a glass or bowl.

2. Drizzle honey on top.

3. If preferred, top with granola for crunch.

4. Continue layering as desired.

5. Indulge in a delicious and filling parfait.

(Preparation time: 5 minutes)

2. Smoothie with Chocolate and Banana

Ingredients:

- Unsweetened cocoa powder - Ripe bananas
- Milk made from almonds
- Optional honey - Ice cubes

Instructions:

1. Blend together ripe bananas, chocolate powder, almond milk, honey (if using), and ice cubes in a blender.

2. Blend until the mixture is smooth and creamy.

3. Pour into a glass and enjoy a chocolaty treat.

(Preparation time: 5 minutes)

3. Almond Butter Apple Slices

Ingredients:

- Almond butter

- Apple slices

- Optional cinnamon

Instructions:

1. Spread almond butter on slices of apple.

2. If preferred, sprinkle with a pinch of cinnamon.

3. Indulge in a quick and nutritious sweet treat.

(Preparation time: 5 minutes)

4. Chia Seed Pudding with Berries

Ingredients:

- Chia seeds and almond milk

- Fresh berries (blueberries, raspberries, etc.)

- Optional: honey

Instructions:

1. Combine chia seeds and almond milk in a jar or container.

2. Stir thoroughly and place in the refrigerator for at least 2 hours or overnight, until thickened.

3. Garnish with fresh berries and sprinkle with honey.

4. Indulge in a healthy chia seed pudding.

(Preparation time: 2 hours or overnight soaking)

5. Date and Almond Energy Balls

Ingredients:

- Almonds, pitted Medjool dates, unsweetened shredded coconut, unsweetened cocoa powder
- Vanilla extract (optional)
- Salt

Instructions:

1. Combine almonds, pitted dates, shredded coconut, cocoa powder, vanilla essence, and a bit of salt (if desired) in a food processor.

2. Process the mixture until it is well mixed and sticky.

3. Make small energy balls out of the mixture.

4. Chill for about 30 minutes in the refrigerator.

5. Enjoy these nutty and sweet goodies.

(Preparation time: 20 minutes)

6. Banana Pops from Frozen

Ingredients:

- Bananas ripe
- Greek yogurt
- Optional: honey
- Chopped nuts (almonds, walnuts, etc.)
- Optional dark chocolate chips

Instructions:

1. Slice ripe bananas in half.

2. Insert a popsicle stick into each side of a banana.

3. Drizzle with honey (if desired), then wrap in chopped nuts or dark chocolate chips (if using).

4. Place on a dish and place in the freezer until solid.

5. Have fun with these frozen banana pops.

(Time to prepare: 15 minutes, including freezing time)

7. Smoothie with Mango and Pineapple

Ingredients:

- Fresh pineapple chunks - Fresh mango chunks
- Cocoa milk
- Optional honey
- Ice cubes

Instructions:

1. Combine mango pieces, pineapple chunks, coconut milk, honey (if using), and ice cubes in a blender.

2. Blend until the mixture is smooth and pleasant.

3. Pour into a glass and enjoy a refreshing tropical smoothie.

(Preparation time: 5 minutes)

8. Cinnamon-Baked Apples

Ingredients:

- Chopped nuts (e.g., walnuts)
- Apples
- Cinnamon
- Honey
- Raisins, if desired

Instructions:

1. Preheat the oven to 375 degrees Fahrenheit (190 degrees Celsius).

2. Peel and core the apples, then cut them into rings or halves.

3. Arrange the apple slices in a baking pan.

4. Drizzle with honey and top with cinnamon-spiced nuts and raisins (if using).

5. Bake for 20-25 minutes, or until the apples are soft.

6. Serve warm for a warm, naturally sweet dessert.

(Preparation time: 30 minutes)

9. Dark Chocolate-Dipped Strawberries

Ingredients:

- Strawberries, fresh

- 70% cacao or higher dark chocolate

- Chopped nuts (such as almonds)

- Optional coconut flakes

Instructions:

1. In a microwave or on the stovetop, melt dark chocolate.

2. Dip each strawberry in melted chocolate before rolling in chopped nuts or coconut flakes (if using).

3. Place on a tray lined with parchment paper.

4. Allow the chocolate to firm and cool.

5. Savor these decadent chocolate-dipped strawberries.

(Preparation time: 15 minutes)

10. Mango Sorbet

Ingredients:

- Peeled and sliced ripe mangoes

- Lime juice

- Optional: honey

Instructions:

1. In a blender, combine diced mangoes.

2. Stir in the lime juice and honey (if using).

3. Puree until smooth.

4. Transfer the mixture to a shallow dish and place in the freezer for about 2-3 hours, stirring occasionally.

5. Serve as a fruity and delightful sorbet.

(Time to prepare: 10 minutes plus freezing time)

10 Beverages

1. Mint Green Tea

Ingredients:

- Bags of green tea

- Mint leaves

- Hot water

Instructions:

1. In a cup, place a green tea bag.

2. Pour in some boiling water and soak for a few minutes.

3. Season with fresh mint leaves.

4. Remove the tea bag and enjoy a cup of calming green tea.

(Preparation time: 5 minutes)

2. Smoothie with blueberries and spinach

Ingredients:

- Blueberries, fresh or frozen
- Fresh spinach leaves
- Greek yogurt
- Optional honey
- Ice cubes

Instructions:

1. Blend together blueberries, spinach, Greek yogurt, honey (if using), and ice cubes in a blender.

2. Blend until the mixture is smooth and vivid.

3. Pour into a glass and enjoy a healthy and refreshing smoothie.

(Preparation time: 5 minutes)

3. Water with Ginger and Lemon Infusion

Ingredients:

- Slices of fresh ginger
- Lemon slices
- Water

Instructions:

1. Fill a pitcher halfway with water.

2. Garnish with fresh ginger and lemon slices.

3. Refrigerate for several hours or overnight to let the flavors to meld.

4. Pour into a glass and enjoy a refreshing and hydrating drink.

(Preparation time: 5 minutes + infusion time)

4. Almond Milk Iced Coffee

Ingredients:

- Unsweetened almond milk
- Cold-brewed coffee
- Sweetener (e.g., agave syrup, honey, or a sugar substitute)
- Ice cubes

Instructions:

1. Combine cold-brewed coffee, unsweetened almond milk, and ice cubes in a glass.

2. If desired, add sweetener to taste.

3. Stir thoroughly and enjoy a nice iced coffee.

(Preparation time: 5 minutes)

5. Watermelon and Mint Cooler

Ingredients:

- Slices of fresh watermelon
- Mint leaves
- Lime juice
- Cubes of ice

Instructions:

1. Blend together watermelon chunks, fresh mint leaves, lime juice, and ice cubes in a blender.

2. Blend until the mixture is smooth and pleasant.

3. Pour into a glass and enjoy a refreshing beverage.

(Preparation time: 5 minutes)

6. Smoothie with Pineapple and Coconut

Ingredients:

- Pineapple chunks, fresh
- Coconut milk
- Yogurt from Greece
- Optional honey
- Ice cubes

Instructions:

1. Blend pineapple pieces, coconut milk, Greek yogurt, honey (if using), and ice cubes in a blender.

2. Puree until smooth and tropical.

3. Strain into a glass and enjoy a refreshing pineapple and coconut smoothie.

(Preparation time: 5 minutes)

7. Water with Lemon and Cucumber

Ingredients:

- Cucumber slices
- Lemon slices
- Water

Instructions:

1. Fill a pitcher halfway with water.

2. Add the lemon and cucumber slices.

3. Refrigerate for several hours or overnight to let the flavors to meld.

4. Pour into a glass and enjoy a pleasant, purifying drink.

(Preparation time: 5 minutes + infusion time)

8. Strawberry Lemonade from scratch

Ingredients:

- Strawberries

- Lemon juice

- Ice cubes

- Water

- Honey (optional)

Instructions:

1. Combine fresh strawberries, lemon juice, water, and honey (if using) in a blender.

2. Puree until smooth.

3. Serve with ice cubes in a glass for a sweet and tart homemade lemonade.

(Preparation time: 10 minutes)

9. Citrus Iced Green Tea

Ingredients:

- Bags of green tea

- Lemon and orange slices

- Warm water

- Cubes of ice

Instructions:

1. Fill a pitcher halfway with green tea bags.

2. Pour in some boiling water and soak for a few minutes.

3. Garnish with lemon and orange slices.

4. Chill until completely cold.

5. Pour over ice to make a delicious, antioxidant-rich iced green tea.

(Preparation time: 10 minutes + chilling time)

10. Smoothie with Beets and Berries

Ingredients:

- Chopped cooked beets
- Mixed berries (strawberries, raspberries)
- Greek yogurt
- Optional honey
- Ice cubes

Instructions:

1. Blend cooked beets, mixed berries, Greek yogurt, honey (if using), and ice cubes in a blender.

2. Blend the mixture until it is vivid and smooth.

3. Serve a bright and nutritious beet and berry smoothie in a glass.

(Preparation time: 5 minutes)

Enjoy!

Conclusion

Finally, the "**Blood Type B+ Diet:** Nourishing Your Body, Your Way" journey of discovery and change has provided you with the information and resources to embrace a healthier and more balanced existence. We've studied the ideas and recommendations suited specifically to Blood Type B+ persons throughout this book, allowing you to harness the power of individualized nutrition.

You've learned how to make intelligent food choices that compliment your specific blood type as you've read through these pages. The accompanying recipes and meal plans not only nourished your body but also suited to your personal preferences, providing a joyful and rewarding culinary experience.

We hope you've noticed a beneficial impact from these dietary modifications, whether it's enhanced vigor, better digestion, weight management, or overall well-being. You've taken a huge step toward a healthier and happier you by following the Blood Type B+ diet.

Keep in mind that your adventure does not finish here. This book's ideas and recipes will continue to assist you on your path to optimal health and energy. We invite you to investigate, experiment, and enjoy the long-term benefits of this tailored nutritional strategy. Your health is valuable, and your future self will be grateful for the investment you've made in your health.

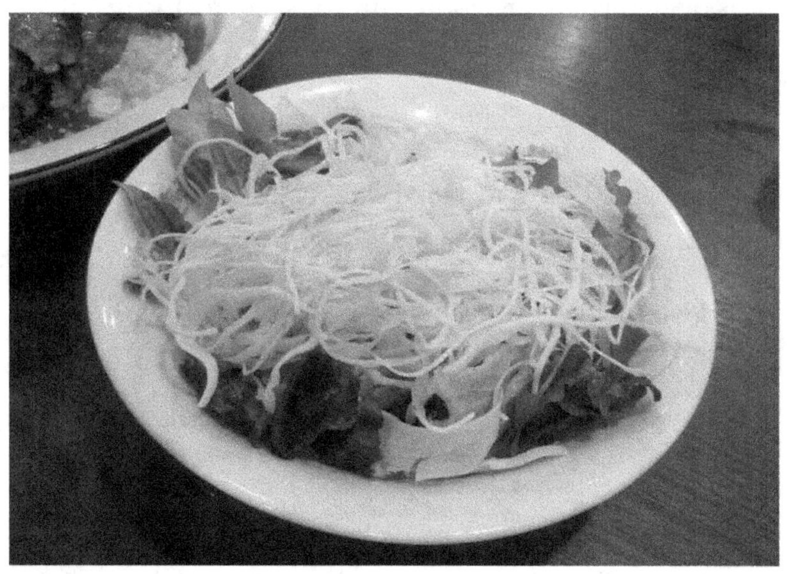

<u>My Little Request</u>

Please take a moment to evaluate my Blood Type B-Positive Diet Book with **FIVE STARS** on Amazon and leave a positive comment if you have appreciated it, dear valued customer. I really value your positive review since it inspired me to write better books.

Thanks!

Journals to Plan Your Diet

B+ FOODS PLANNER

MONDAY	BREAKFAST	
	LUNCH	
	DINNER	
TUESDAY	BREAKFAST	
	LUNCH	
	DINNER	
WEDNESDAY	BREAKFAST	
	LUNCH	
	DINNER	
THURSDAY	BREAKFAST	
	LUNCH	
	DINNER	
FRIDAY	BREAKFAST	
	LUNCH	
	DINNER	
SATURDAY	BREAKFAST	
	LUNCH	
	DINNER	
SUNDAY	BREAKFAST	
	LUNCH	
	DINNER	

GROCERY LIST

SNACKS

B+ FOODS PLANNER

MONDAY	BREAKFAST	
	LUNCH	
	DINNER	
TUESDAY	BREAKFAST	
	LUNCH	
	DINNER	
WEDNESDAY	BREAKFAST	
	LUNCH	
	DINNER	
THURSDAY	BREAKFAST	
	LUNCH	
	DINNER	
FRIDAY	BREAKFAST	
	LUNCH	
	DINNER	
SATURDAY	BREAKFAST	
	LUNCH	
	DINNER	
SUNDAY	BREAKFAST	
	LUNCH	
	DINNER	

GROCERY LIST

SNACKS

B+ FOODS PLANNER

			GROCERY LIST
MONDAY	BREAKFAST		
	LUNCH		
	DINNER		
TUESDAY	BREAKFAST		
	LUNCH		
	DINNER		
WEDNESDAY	BREAKFAST		
	LUNCH		
	DINNER		
THURSDAY	BREAKFAST		
	LUNCH		
	DINNER		
FRIDAY	BREAKFAST		SNACKS
	LUNCH		
	DINNER		
SATURDAY	BREAKFAST		
	LUNCH		
	DINNER		
SUNDAY	BREAKFAST		
	LUNCH		
	DINNER		

B+ FOODS PLANNER

MONDAY	BREAKFAST	
	LUNCH	
	DINNER	
TUESDAY	BREAKFAST	
	LUNCH	
	DINNER	
WEDNESDAY	BREAKFAST	
	LUNCH	
	DINNER	
THURSDAY	BREAKFAST	
	LUNCH	
	DINNER	
FRIDAY	BREAKFAST	
	LUNCH	
	DINNER	
SATURDAY	BREAKFAST	
	LUNCH	
	DINNER	
SUNDAY	BREAKFAST	
	LUNCH	
	DINNER	

GROCERY LIST

SNACKS

B+ FOODS PLANNER

MONDAY	BREAKFAST	
	LUNCH	
	DINNER	
TUESDAY	BREAKFAST	
	LUNCH	
	DINNER	
WEDNESDAY	BREAKFAST	
	LUNCH	
	DINNER	
THURSDAY	BREAKFAST	
	LUNCH	
	DINNER	
FRIDAY	BREAKFAST	
	LUNCH	
	DINNER	
SATURDAY	BREAKFAST	
	LUNCH	
	DINNER	
SUNDAY	BREAKFAST	
	LUNCH	
	DINNER	

GROCERY LIST

SNACKS

B+ FOODS PLANNER

MONDAY	BREAKFAST	
	LUNCH	
	DINNER	
TUESDAY	BREAKFAST	
	LUNCH	
	DINNER	
WEDNESDAY	BREAKFAST	
	LUNCH	
	DINNER	
THURSDAY	BREAKFAST	
	LUNCH	
	DINNER	
FRIDAY	BREAKFAST	
	LUNCH	
	DINNER	
SATURDAY	BREAKFAST	
	LUNCH	
	DINNER	
SUNDAY	BREAKFAST	
	LUNCH	
	DINNER	

GROCERY LIST

SNACKS

B+ FOODS PLANNER

MONDAY	BREAKFAST	
	LUNCH	
	DINNER	
TUESDAY	BREAKFAST	
	LUNCH	
	DINNER	
WEDNESDAY	BREAKFAST	
	LUNCH	
	DINNER	
THURSDAY	BREAKFAST	
	LUNCH	
	DINNER	
FRIDAY	BREAKFAST	
	LUNCH	
	DINNER	
SATURDAY	BREAKFAST	
	LUNCH	
	DINNER	
SUNDAY	BREAKFAST	
	LUNCH	
	DINNER	

GROCERY LIST

SNACKS

B+ FOODS PLANNER

			GROCERY LIST
MONDAY	BREAKFAST		
	LUNCH		
	DINNER		
TUESDAY	BREAKFAST		
	LUNCH		
	DINNER		
WEDNESDAY	BREAKFAST		
	LUNCH		
	DINNER		
THURSDAY	BREAKFAST		
	LUNCH		
	DINNER		
FRIDAY	BREAKFAST		SNACKS
	LUNCH		
	DINNER		
SATURDAY	BREAKFAST		
	LUNCH		
	DINNER		
SUNDAY	BREAKFAST		
	LUNCH		
	DINNER		

B+ FOODS PLANNER

			GROCERY LIST
MONDAY	BREAKFAST		
	LUNCH		
	DINNER		
TUESDAY	BREAKFAST		
	LUNCH		
	DINNER		
WEDNESDAY	BREAKFAST		
	LUNCH		
	DINNER		
THURSDAY	BREAKFAST		
	LUNCH		
	DINNER		
FRIDAY	BREAKFAST		SNACKS
	LUNCH		
	DINNER		
SATURDAY	BREAKFAST		
	LUNCH		
	DINNER		
SUNDAY	BREAKFAST		
	LUNCH		
	DINNER		

B+ FOODS PLANNER

MONDAY	BREAKFAST	
	LUNCH	
	DINNER	
TUESDAY	BREAKFAST	
	LUNCH	
	DINNER	
WEDNESDAY	BREAKFAST	
	LUNCH	
	DINNER	
THURSDAY	BREAKFAST	
	LUNCH	
	DINNER	
FRIDAY	BREAKFAST	
	LUNCH	
	DINNER	
SATURDAY	BREAKFAST	
	LUNCH	
	DINNER	
SUNDAY	BREAKFAST	
	LUNCH	
	DINNER	

GROCERY LIST

SNACKS

B+ FOODS PLANNER

MONDAY	BREAKFAST	
	LUNCH	
	DINNER	
TUESDAY	BREAKFAST	
	LUNCH	
	DINNER	
WEDNESDAY	BREAKFAST	
	LUNCH	
	DINNER	
THURSDAY	BREAKFAST	
	LUNCH	
	DINNER	
FRIDAY	BREAKFAST	
	LUNCH	
	DINNER	
SATURDAY	BREAKFAST	
	LUNCH	
	DINNER	
SUNDAY	BREAKFAST	
	LUNCH	
	DINNER	

GROCERY LIST

SNACKS

B+ FOODS PLANNER

MONDAY	BREAKFAST	
	LUNCH	
	DINNER	
TUESDAY	BREAKFAST	
	LUNCH	
	DINNER	
WEDNESDAY	BREAKFAST	
	LUNCH	
	DINNER	
THURSDAY	BREAKFAST	
	LUNCH	
	DINNER	
FRIDAY	BREAKFAST	
	LUNCH	
	DINNER	
SATURDAY	BREAKFAST	
	LUNCH	
	DINNER	
SUNDAY	BREAKFAST	
	LUNCH	
	DINNER	

GROCERY LIST

SNACKS

B+ FOODS PLANNER

MONDAY	BREAKFAST	
	LUNCH	
	DINNER	
TUESDAY	BREAKFAST	
	LUNCH	
	DINNER	
WEDNESDAY	BREAKFAST	
	LUNCH	
	DINNER	
THURSDAY	BREAKFAST	
	LUNCH	
	DINNER	
FRIDAY	BREAKFAST	
	LUNCH	
	DINNER	
SATURDAY	BREAKFAST	
	LUNCH	
	DINNER	
SUNDAY	BREAKFAST	
	LUNCH	
	DINNER	

GROCERY LIST

SNACKS

B+ FOODS PLANNER

MONDAY	BREAKFAST	
	LUNCH	
	DINNER	
TUESDAY	BREAKFAST	
	LUNCH	
	DINNER	
WEDNESDAY	BREAKFAST	
	LUNCH	
	DINNER	
THURSDAY	BREAKFAST	
	LUNCH	
	DINNER	
FRIDAY	BREAKFAST	
	LUNCH	
	DINNER	
SATURDAY	BREAKFAST	
	LUNCH	
	DINNER	
SUNDAY	BREAKFAST	
	LUNCH	
	DINNER	

GROCERY LIST

SNACKS

B+ FOODS PLANNER

			GROCERY LIST
MONDAY	BREAKFAST		
	LUNCH		
	DINNER		
TUESDAY	BREAKFAST		
	LUNCH		
	DINNER		
WEDNESDAY	BREAKFAST		
	LUNCH		
	DINNER		
THURSDAY	BREAKFAST		
	LUNCH		
	DINNER		
FRIDAY	BREAKFAST		SNACKS
	LUNCH		
	DINNER		
SATURDAY	BREAKFAST		
	LUNCH		
	DINNER		
SUNDAY	BREAKFAST		
	LUNCH		
	DINNER		

B+ FOODS PLANNER

MONDAY	BREAKFAST	
	LUNCH	
	DINNER	
TUESDAY	BREAKFAST	
	LUNCH	
	DINNER	
WEDNESDAY	BREAKFAST	
	LUNCH	
	DINNER	
THURSDAY	BREAKFAST	
	LUNCH	
	DINNER	
FRIDAY	BREAKFAST	
	LUNCH	
	DINNER	
SATURDAY	BREAKFAST	
	LUNCH	
	DINNER	
SUNDAY	BREAKFAST	
	LUNCH	
	DINNER	

GROCERY LIST

SNACKS

B+ FOODS PLANNER

MONDAY	BREAKFAST	
	LUNCH	
	DINNER	
TUESDAY	BREAKFAST	
	LUNCH	
	DINNER	
WEDNESDAY	BREAKFAST	
	LUNCH	
	DINNER	
THURSDAY	BREAKFAST	
	LUNCH	
	DINNER	
FRIDAY	BREAKFAST	
	LUNCH	
	DINNER	
SATURDAY	BREAKFAST	
	LUNCH	
	DINNER	
SUNDAY	BREAKFAST	
	LUNCH	
	DINNER	

GROCERY LIST

SNACKS

B+ FOODS PLANNER

			GROCERY LIST
MONDAY	BREAKFAST		
	LUNCH		
	DINNER		
TUESDAY	BREAKFAST		
	LUNCH		
	DINNER		
WEDNESDAY	BREAKFAST		
	LUNCH		
	DINNER		
THURSDAY	BREAKFAST		
	LUNCH		
	DINNER		
FRIDAY	BREAKFAST		
	LUNCH		SNACKS
	DINNER		
SATURDAY	BREAKFAST		
	LUNCH		
	DINNER		
SUNDAY	BREAKFAST		
	LUNCH		
	DINNER		

B+ FOODS PLANNER

MONDAY	BREAKFAST	
	LUNCH	
	DINNER	
TUESDAY	BREAKFAST	
	LUNCH	
	DINNER	
WEDNESDAY	BREAKFAST	
	LUNCH	
	DINNER	
THURSDAY	BREAKFAST	
	LUNCH	
	DINNER	
FRIDAY	BREAKFAST	
	LUNCH	
	DINNER	
SATURDAY	BREAKFAST	
	LUNCH	
	DINNER	
SUNDAY	BREAKFAST	
	LUNCH	
	DINNER	

GROCERY LIST

SNACKS

B+ FOODS PLANNER

			GROCERY LIST
MONDAY	BREAKFAST		
	LUNCH		
	DINNER		
TUESDAY	BREAKFAST		
	LUNCH		
	DINNER		
WEDNESDAY	BREAKFAST		
	LUNCH		
	DINNER		
THURSDAY	BREAKFAST		
	LUNCH		
	DINNER		
FRIDAY	BREAKFAST		SNACKS
	LUNCH		
	DINNER		
SATURDAY	BREAKFAST		
	LUNCH		
	DINNER		
SUNDAY	BREAKFAST		
	LUNCH		
	DINNER		

www.ingramcontent.com/pod-product-compliance
Lightning Source LLC
Chambersburg PA
CBHW050835260726

48660CB00006B/2255